Antimicrobial Resistance
and One-Health Approaches

Antimicrobial Resistance and One-Health Approaches

Ramendra Pandey
Arpana Vibhuti
Chung-Ming Chang

ELIVA PRESS

Published by Eliva Press
Email: info@elivapress.com
Website: www.elivapress.com

ISBN: 978-1-63648-336-8

© Eliva Press, 2021
© Ramendra Pandey, Arpana Vibhuti, Chung-Ming Chang
Cover Design: Eliva Press
Cover Image: Freepik Premium
Printed at: see last page

One Health

Riya Mukherjee[1], Ramendra Pati Pandey[1]*, Chung-Ming Chang[2]*

Centre for Drug Design Discovery and Development (C4D), SRM University, Delhi-NCR, Rajiv Gandhi Education City, Sonepat - 131 029, Haryana, India;

[2]Master & Ph.D. program in Biotechnology Industry, Chang Gung University, No.259, Wenhua 1st Rd., Guishan Dist. Taoyuan City 33302, Taiwan (R.O.C.);

*Corresponding authors:

Chung-Ming Chang*, Master & Ph.D. program in Biotechnology Industry, Chang Gung University, No.259, Wenhua 1st Rd., Guishan Dist. Taoyuan City 33302, Taiwan (R.O.C.),

Ramendra Pati Pandey*, Centre for Drug Design Discovery and Development (C4D), SRM University, Delhi-NCR, Rajiv Gandhi Education City, Sonepat - 131 029, Haryana, India

Contents

Summary

This chapter brings in the introduction to this newly expanded field of One Health. In addition, the chapter elucidates a significant approach for attaining optimal health care for the people along with that, this benefits the reader by acknowledging them with the following points.

- ❖ A thorough explanation of One Health.
- ❖ Why there is a need of One Health Approach?
- ❖ How this approach works?
- ❖ Provides an overview of One Health through the different disciplines.

Also includes different applications of One Health Approach.

In the text "On Airs, Waters, and Places" written by the Greek Physician Hippocrates mentioned that the health of the humankind completely depends on the environment. As long as the environment is clean, health of the humans will be under check and can be controlled. Moreover, the Veterinary Public Health Division at the Centers for Disease Control and Prevention (CDC) contributed in explaining the possibility of transmission of diseases among the animals and human. (1) In addition, it has provided detailed information about the epidemiology of zoonotic diseases. Thus, this prospect opens up the burgeoning domain of One Health. One Health is considered to be the transdisciplinary approach wherein multiple sectors come together to achieve better optimal health outcomes. This approach is worked at local, national and in global stages that aids in understanding the interconnected relation among animals, plants and their common shared environment. The special concept of One Health calls attention to the interconnection of human health with the health of animals and environment. This whole approach is of great importance because of the emerging contagious zoonotic diseases. According to the studies, the contagious diseases among humans are found to be 65% zoonotic

3

diseases. Thus, to understand the epidemiology and etiology, multiple sectors are required for achieving better results in generating optimal health outcomes. There is a prominent increase in the number of epidemics and zoonoses globally. Moreover, this rapid spread of zoonoses and epidemics, increased the menace of pandemic worldwide. There are various components that have impelled the nature by manifesting how important role is played by the animal and human ecosystem in emergence of newly diverse organisms and in evolution of the planet. It is extremely important to integrate the human, animal, plant health with biodiversity to understand the statistics of emergence of various infectious diseases globally along with the concerns escalated by the antimicrobial resistance, environmental pollution and many other artificial outcomes. These are the major challenges that are faced by the humankind which requires immediate attention so as to reduce the number of epidemics and pandemics. (2) The diagram

below demonstrates how the integration of the three health is crucial to develop this One Health Approach for improving the health outcomes in future research. (**Figure 1**)

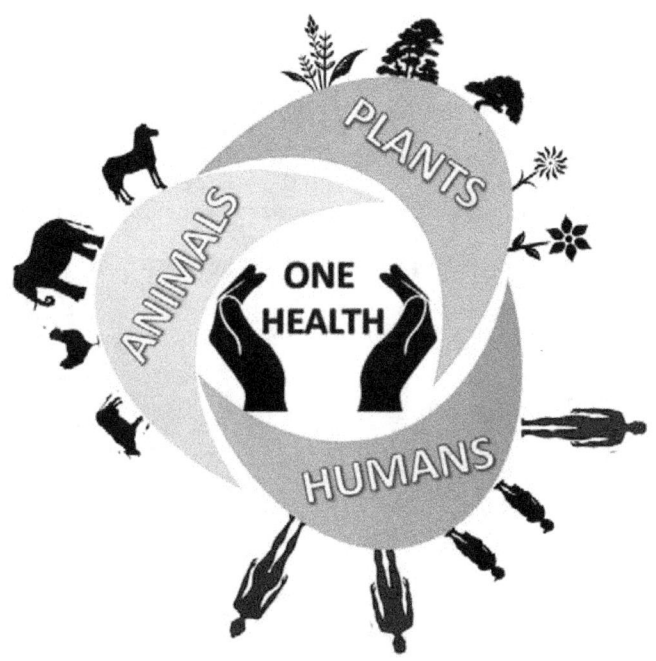

Figure 1. Integration of Plant Health, Animal Health and Human Health to initiate the One Health Approach globally.

What We Know About One Health?

One Health Approach facilitates this interdisciplinary indulgence to control the emergence of the diseases and is advantageous in helping to put a check on the existing diseases. This approach will strategically consider all the problems that are arising due to the emerging and existing diseases and will effectively provide a detailed information about the outcomes or updates. One of the major issues, emergence of antimicrobial resistance is also being addressed through this One Health Approach. We all require a better acknowledgement about the consequences along with the causes of the human activities, their lifestyles and their doings for the environment in the ecosystem as these are crucial to interpret the disease drift. **(Figure 2)** (2, 3) Therefore, the amelioration of the globe is in understanding all the aspects clearly on a global scale and integration of all the health together for fighting against the challenges powerfully.

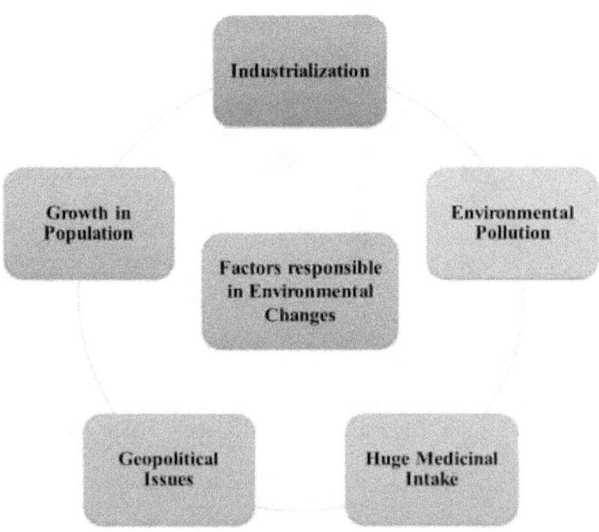

Figure 2. Human Activities actively responsible in environmental changes globally

Interestingly, One Health Approach is an old concept which was previously termed as "One Medicine" that supported the combination of various human medicines and veterinary medicines to combat the zoonotic diseases. Later on in the year 2004, the concept for One Health appeared, which was an initiative to incorporate all the three health aspects for making it a multidisciplinary expertise to deal with animals, humans, plants and their shared ecosystem. (4) (**Figure 3**) Initially, this concept was stuck with the zoonotic diseases and the medicines towards those but eventually the One Health Approach is opening up in other respects such as antimicrobial resistance, toxicology or other health habits in the environment. Hence, One Health proves to be an effective approach both for infectious diseases as well as non-infectious diseases.

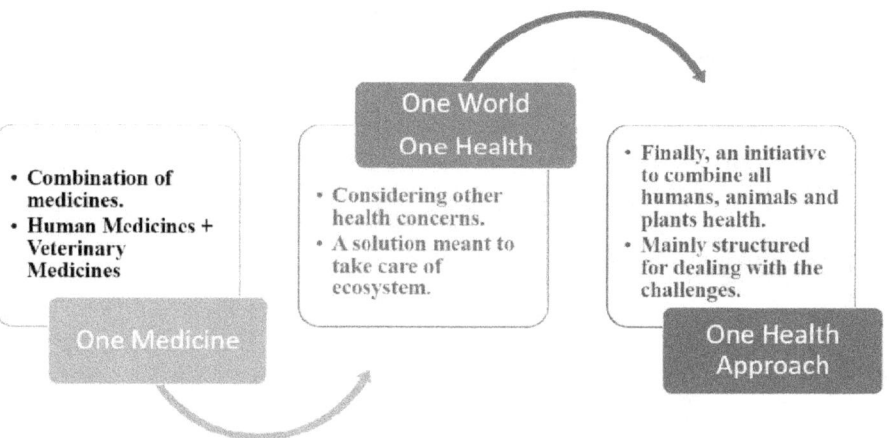

Figure 3. The process of One Health Approach Initiative

Why there is need for One Health Approach?

In the beginning of the chapter, it is raised that One Health Approach is not a new topic instead has become focus of attention due to its importance in the recent years. This has been more prominent due to several factors of environment and humankind which have changed the major interactions among each individual in the ecosystem. (**Figure 4**)

Over the period of time, there has been huge climatic change in the Earth. The Earth has experienced huge loss in terms of deforestation and many other human activities which have led in the emergence of imbalance in the ecosystem.

Massive industrialization and urbanization have been proved to be disadvantageous for the nature due to immense pollution.

Growth in human population is another major concern for the environment. More the number of human populations more are the usage of land thereby destroying massive areas.

Moreover, the expand in the human populations have brought the animals in close contact with the humans as animals play a vital role in human's lives. Through livestock or pets, the microorganisms can easily make their way to humans.

Trading across the globe for multiple commodities have spread the transmission of diseases very easily.

Due to the intake of innumerable medicines for the diseases, antimicrobial resistance has emerged massively.

All these aforementioned issues have made the One Health Approach, one of the important aspects in the life science research. (5, 6) So, the common issues that are hoped to be resolved by this One Health Approach are emerging antimicrobial resistance, new emerging and existing zoonotic diseases, environmental contamination, vector-borne diseases and many other threats related to health which are interconnected among animals, humans and plants. All these elements have proved to be the reason behind the increasing number of epidemics, endemics and pandemics worldwide. (6)

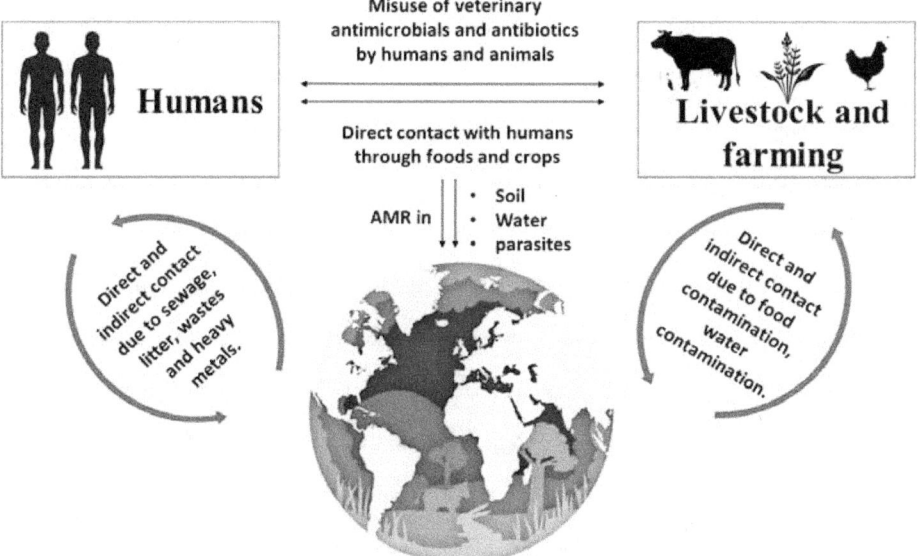

Figure 4. The conceptual diagram depicts several factors for transmission of the diseases in the ecosystem. AMR: Antimicrobial Resistance.

Working Mechanism of One Health Approach

As One Health Approach involves multidisciplinary sectors thus, experts who are active in different sectors join altogether such as human health (nurses, doctors, epidemiologists), animal health (veterinarians, agricultural workers), environment (wildlife experts, ecologists) and many other areas of expertise meet up to coordinate with their activities. (**Figure 5**) The whole mechanism of One Health Approach does not comprise of one individual, organization or sector instead a bunch of professionals can address the never-ending issues related to health. Therefore, relevant experts from different disciplines can contribute in delivering the best results or strategies against the emerging issues. (7) These are studied thoroughly from different other perspectives and later on the conclusion is drawn from their study. Some of the eminent organizations such as American Veterinary Medical Association, American Medical Association, Centers for Disease Control and Prevention, United States Department of Agriculture have come forward to be the part of this initiative. A huge effectiveness has been found in the collaboration of FAO, OIE and WHO (Food and Agriculture Organization, World Organization for Animal Health, World Health Organization) for implementing the One Health Approach principles internationally. (8, 9) (1)However, a distinguished involvement of many regions especially developing countries are also taking this One Health initiative seriously and are putting all efforts to the extent of their own capabilities. (10)It is very important to understand that, to effectively have the surveillance, detection, response and to prevent the probable outbreaks of the diseases and other food safety issues, relevant data such as epidemiological data, laboratory information needs to be shared all across the respective departments, be it national, local, regional or global levels. The intervention of these respective levels aids in the implementation of the responses jointly taken against the health threats. (3, 11)

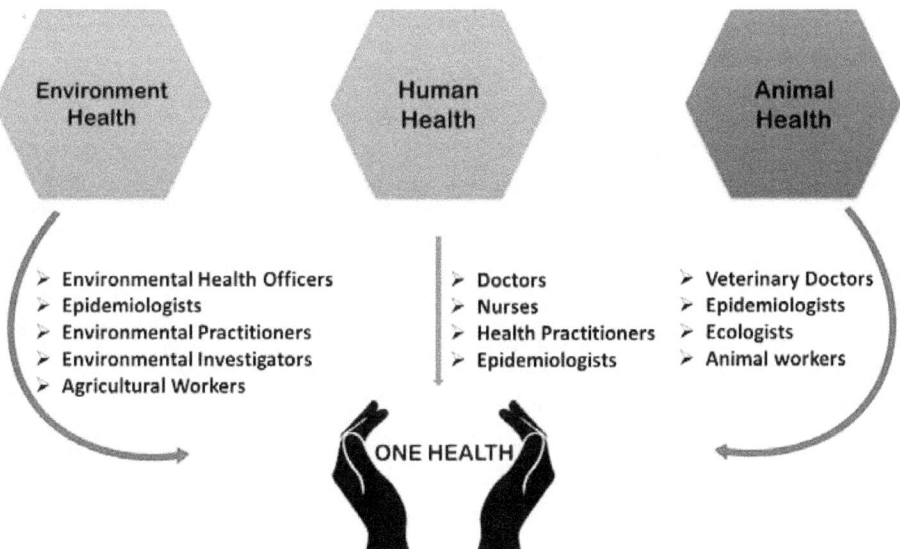

Figure 5. One Health Approach, a multidisciplinary approach consisting different experts from various fields.

Despite the involvement of various professionals, many other experts from different field also needs equal attention for this approach. There are many core competency domains for One Health Approach and surprisingly, both Global Health Domains and One Health domains cooperate to contribute in resolving the common issues related to animal and human ecosystem. **(Figure 6.)** The purpose is to use the strategic evaluations to strategically analyze the diverse form of range in terms of interrelated elements that proves to contribute in increase the complexity more. (11, 12)

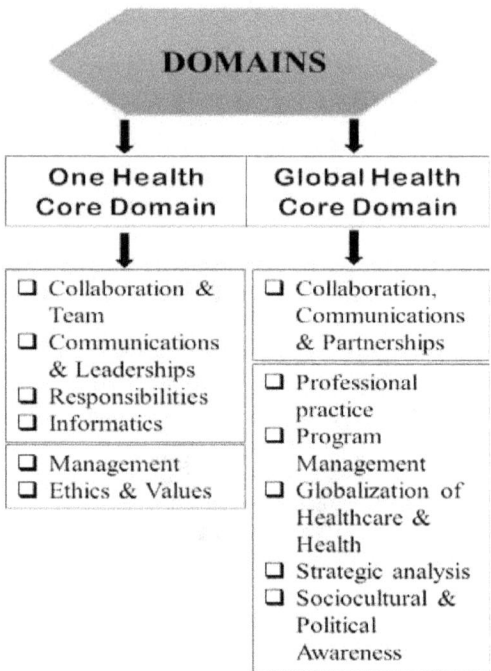

Figure 6. The conceptual flowchart mentions the other domains equally participating in the One Health Approach Initiative.

Application of One Health Approach

Until now we came across the term 'collaboration' which is required for this One Health concept to work. And this collaboration of various disciplines worldwide is needed for setting up the protocols and policies so as to understand the necessary elements that require huge attention to figure out the relatedness with the occurrence of any specific disease. For example, the case of leptospirosis was found to be related with various factors like socioeconomic factors (Sanitation, Poverty, Impoverished Housing Conditions), Number of animals by property, soil type, land use, etc. Similarly, studies on the cases of yellow fiver have been found to be related on environmental as well as geographic factors. The context of application is further subdivided into three segments for making it easy for the readers to understand the application of One Health Concept. (**Figure 7**)(11, 13, 14)

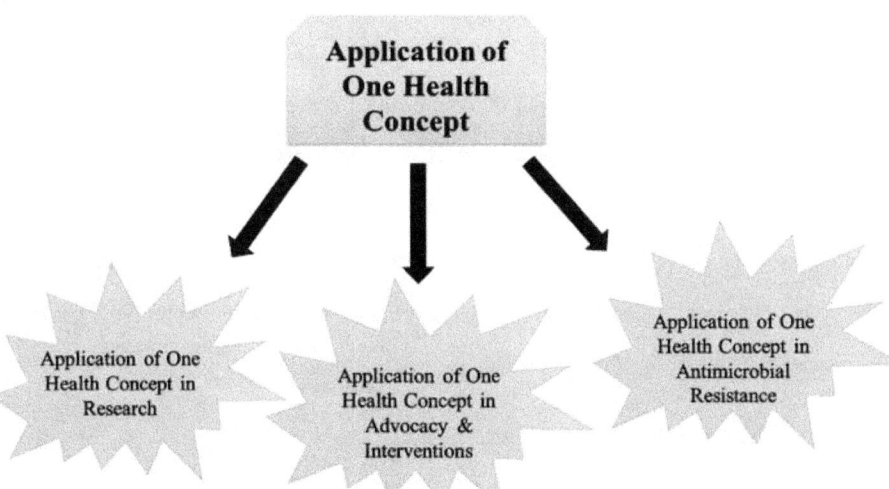

Figure 7. Application of One Health Approach

1. **Application in Research**

One Health Research requires data for humans, animals and environment to relate among each other for the better outcomes. More number of research are done in this field to predict the possibilities and prepare accordingly for facing the hurdles. Massive pathogens spillover is everywhere due to several human activities and to understand the whole process One Health Concept is in great use in research field. It will not only help in finding out the source for the emergence but also will help in predicting other criteria to deliver impactful and effective response. The whole process of the etiology of the pathogen, the mechanism of the transmission of the particular pathogen, the spillover of the disease everywhere causing either epidemics or pandemics can be closely studied through the research. This requires collaborative work for acquiring potent data that will further help in statistical data analysis for meeting the dots required to observe the impact that the diseases make on the public health. Different models are formed for better understanding of the infection dynamics. For example, mathematical models are used as a tool for the application of One Health Concept as this helps in reducing the complexity which rises because of the life cycles and transmission process of the pathogens. Moreover, the effect of interventions can be studied through this. One of the examples where the One Health Approach is quite in use is in the case of SARS (severe acute respiratory syndrome) and Avian Influenza where the collaborative work was required for improve the quality of monitoring from all aspects for better health outcomes in future.(11, 15, 16)

2. Application in Advocacy and Interventions

Several researches support the use of the One Health strategy in tickborne pathogen therapies. The rise in human cases of avian influenza H5N1 in Asia in 2006, as well as the risk of transmission to other areas of the world, highlighted the looming threat of pandemics and the significance of cross-sector collaboration. In order to organize solutions, an integrated vision was required. Thus, migratory wild birds may come into touch with influenza virus and spread it to other domestic animals and humans. Furthermore, a greater understanding of how people, products, and trade interact is critical for global security; for example, the clear risk of markets with high animal density and insufficient biosafety, as well as the extensive production of birds, and different animal products. It is critical to strengthen surveillance across sectors, share information, and develop new techniques. The development of pandemic prevention measures through cross-sector collaboration was an excellent exercise in coherent understanding and effort—as well as preparedness for any zoonotic disease disaster. A One Health study examined human yellow fever cases and discovered that geographic patterns and environmental factors were related to altitude, rainfall, temperature, and the diversity of nonhuman primate hosts.(11, 17)

3. Application in AMR (Antimicrobial Resistance)

Antimicrobial resistance (AMR) is becoming increasingly important and can only be addressed through the One Health approach. AMR occurs when microorganisms adapt to antimicrobial drugs and become ineffective, letting microorganisms to proliferate. Antibiotics and antimicrobial agents have been an essential part of treating patients with infectious diseases in the past years. The drugs have played a critical role in reducing illness and death. Nonetheless, rampant use of these drugs has come at a cost: the infectious organisms that even the antibiotics are meant to kill have adapted to them, rendering the drugs less effective. Pathogenic bacteria (e.g., *Salmonella spp.*, *Campylobacter spp.*) as well as commensal bacteria (e.g., *E. coli*, *Enterococcus spp.*) can be transmitted from animals to people through food, direct contact with animals, or environmental sources such as contaminated water. (11)The necessity of the One Health concept has been underlined as the overuse of antimicrobials in domestic animal husbandry and its possible consequences on the human population has become more generally acknowledged. AMR is recognized as a major worldwide problem, and various campaigns and organizations around the world are working to raise awareness about it. Furthermore, in order to alleviate the impacts of AMR, these organizations advocate for the safe use of antimicrobials in humans, animals, and the environment. (18)

Conclusion

The chapter explains how important ecological, evolutionary, and environmental studies are in understanding the genesis and re-emergence of infectious and non-communicable chronic diseases, and establishing novel control techniques. Removing the interdisciplinary barriers that still exist between ecological, environmental, and evolutionary sciences and animals and humans medicine is a significant way to implement the "One Health" concept, which extends beyond scientific research and impacts health, agriculture, land management, urbanism, and biological sustainability), law, and ethics. The evidence on the increased value of the "One Health" strategy is needed for governments, researchers, and funding agencies.

References

1. Wikipedia. One Health [Available from: https://en.wikipedia.org/wiki/One_Health.

2. Muringatheri M. One Health concept gains importance The Hindu. 2020 February 16.

3. Prevention CfDCa. One Health Basics

    [Availablefrom:https://www.cdc.gov/onehealth/basics/history/index.html.

4. Delphine Destoumieux-Garzón, Gilles Boetsch, Jérôme Boissier, Frédéric Darriet, Priscilla Duboz, Clémentine Fritsch, Patrick Giraudoux, Frédérique Le Roux, Serge Morand, Christine Paillard, Dominique Pontier, Cédric Sueur, Yann Voituron The One Health Concept: 10 Years Old and a Long Road Ahead. Front Vet Sci. 2018.

5. John S Mackenzie MJ. The One Health Approach—Why Is It So Important? Trop Med Infect Dis. 2019;4(2):88.

6. Sharon L. Deem KEL-d, Elizabeth A. Rayhel. Introduction to One Health: An Interdisciplinary Approach to Planetary Health2018 November 2018.

7.   Catherine Machalaba, Jill Raufman , Assaf Anyamba, Amanda M. Berrian, Franck C. J. Berthe, Gregory C. Gray, et al. Applying a One Health Approach in Global Health and Medicine: Enhancing Involvement of Medical Schools and Global Health Centers. Annals og Global Health.

8.   Health WOFA. One Health [Available from: https://www.oie.int/en/what-we-do/global-initiatives/one-health/.

9.   Jogerst K, Callender, B., Adams, V., Evert, J., Fields, E., Hall, T., . . . Wilson, L. L. . Identifying interprofessional global health competencies for 21st-century health professionals. Annals of Global Health. 2015;81(2):239-7.

10.   Health   WOfa.   [Available   from: https://www.oie.int/en/what-we-do/global-initiatives/one-health/.

11.   Maria Cristina Schneider CM-Z, Kyung-duk Min and Sylvain Aldighieri. "One Health" From Concept to Application in the Global World. Global Public Health. 2019.

12.   Frankson R HW, Christian K, Olson D, Lee M, Valeri L, Hyatt R, Annelli J, Rubin C. One Health Core Competency Domains. . Front Public Health 2016:192.

13.   J Landford 1 MN. Good governance in 'one health' approaches. Rev Sci Tech. 2012;2.

14.   Mackenzie JS MM, Jeggo M. One Health: From Concept to Practice. Confronting Emerging Zoonoses. 2014:163–89.

15.   Kelley Lee ZLB. Operationalizing the One Health approach: the global governance challenges. Health Policy and Planning. 2013;28(7):778-85.

16.   Lisa M Gargano PFG, Meredith Barrett, Kelly Howell, Cameron Wolfe, Christopher Woods, James M Hughes. Issues in the development of a research and education framework for one health. Emerg Infect Dis. 2013.

17.   Bhatia R. Implementation framework for One Health approach. Indian J Med Res. 2019;149((3)):329–31. .

18.   Organization WH. Antimicrobial resistance 2018

Antimicrobial resistance (AMR) and Immune homeostasis

Ramendra Pati Pandey[1], Chung-Ming Chang[2]*

Centre for Drug Design Discovery and Development (C4D), SRM University, Delhi-NCR, Rajiv Gandhi Education City, Sonepat - 131 029, Haryana, India;

[2]Master & Ph.D. program in Biotechnology Industry, Chang Gung University, No.259, Wenhua 1st Rd., Guishan Dist. Taoyuan City 33302, Taiwan (R.O.C.); cmchang@mail.cgu.edu.tw (C.M.C.)

*Corresponding author:

Chung-Ming Chang*, Master & Ph.D. program in Biotechnology Industry, Chang Gung University, No.259, Wenhua 1st Rd., Guishan Dist. Taoyuan City 33302, Taiwan (R.O.C.)

Antimicrobial resistance (AMR) possesses an extreme threat to global health and modern medicine. Antibiotic resistance is rising to dangerously high levels in all parts of the world. Antibiotic resistance leads to higher medical costs, prolonged hospital stays, and increased mortality. The emergence of resistance to last-resort antibiotics is a public health concern of global scale. Antibiotics are overused in treating patients even with coughs and colds that do not require antibiotic treatment. In many places, antibiotics are overused and misused in people and animals, and often given without professional oversight. Drug resistant-microbes are found in people, animals, food, and the environment (in water, soil and air). They can spread between people and animals, and from person to person. Poor infection control, inadequate sanitary conditions and inappropriate food-handling encourage the spread of antimicrobial resistance. So, the World Health Organization sent a red alert to all the member countries to pay immediate attention to all these dangerous pathogens.

Viruses are constantly evolving; many respiratory outbreaks show "flu like" symptoms. A number of modern testing strategies can be used to detect virus in the laboratory like: Genomics, Proteomics, Specific host response profile, immune response pattern, metabolomics and bioinformatics. We can use Hierarchical Clustering method (bioinformatics method) to categorize new viruses. These strategies can be used to meet the epidemiological situation and laboratory capabilities. By the use of these strategies we can distinguish changes in cellular gene expression and protein profiles that occur in response to virus infection. Now is the time to understand virology at a system level by the use of genomic and proteomic tools. There is a very motivating window in the virus research to study virus-host interactions in a more comprehensive manner to discover exciting new insights into immunity, and the strategies used by influenza virus to overcome cellular defenses.

Lactic acid cultures and their fermented products provide therapeutic and nutritional benefits to the consumers (Parvez *et al.* 2006). Organisms used as probiotics majorly include the member of genera *Lactobacillus or Bifidobacterium, Escherichia coli, Bacillus subtilis, Saccharomyces boulardii* and *Enterococcus faecium* (Toole and Cooney 2008). It has been investigated that most of the probiotic strains exhibited common properties but there are differences in their mode of action. These facts signify that probiotic attributes are strain specific and each probiotic strain should be tested individually. The major mode of action includes altering the immune system. Gut microbiota has direct contact with intestinal epithelial cells, which in turn has direct interface with immune system. At intestinal surface, microbes are recognised by receptors on the surface of epithelium, which is a prime activator of immunological response. Bacterial molecular structures like lipopolysaccharides (LPS), lipoteichoic acids and unmethylated CpG DNA motifs are recognised by pattern recognition receptors such as Toll-like receptors. Probiotic bacteria are also known to activate pro-inflammatory cytokines and chemokines (Saxelin *et al.* 2005).

Gut Immune homeostasis:

Interactions between the host immune system and micro flora are important to understand the progression of IBD. In mouse models, it is known that normal flora regulates intestinal immune cell development. Transforming growth factor (TGF)-β and IL-6, plays an essential role in differentiation of Th17 and Treg cells (Stockinger & Veldhoen, 2007). Ivanov et al. revealed that segmented filamentous bacterium (SFB), is enough to induce the appearance of Th17 cells in the lamina propria. The introduction of fecal material from germ free mice colonized with SFB into Jackson B6 mice by oral gavage induced robust Th17 cell differentiation. SFB colonization resulted in reduced growth of an intestinal pathogen, suggesting that intestinal commensal microbes can contribute to Th17 cell-mediated mucosal protection (Ivanov et al., 2009). Atarashi et al. stated that indigenous Clostridium species promote colonic Treg cell accumulation. In mice, it has been found that colonization by a distinct mix of Clostridium strains affected Foxp3$^+$ Treg cell number and function in the colon provided an environment rich in TGF-β (Atarashi et al., 2011). H. hepaticus colonization leads to disease and pro-inflammatory cytokine production in colonic tissues. PSA (Polysaccharide A) is required to suppress pro-inflammatory IL-17 production by intestinal immune cells and protects from inflammatory disease through an IL-10-producing CD4$^+$Treg cell type (Mazmanian et al., 2008). Round et al. revealed that PSA derived from B. fragilis directs the development of Foxp3$^+$T cells. Animals with B. fragilis increase the suppressive capacity of Tregs in the gut (Round & Mazmanian, 2010). Foxp3$^+$Tregs regulate the homeostatic functional property of PSA from B. fragilisis through Toll-like receptor (TLR) 2-dependent signal transduction (Round et al., 2011). TCRs did not facilitate thymic Treg cell development, implying that many colonic Treg cells arise by antigen-specific peripheral education (Barrett et al., 2008). Mice with T-bet deficiency in the innate immune system (T-bet−/− and RAG2−/− mice) developed spontaneous colitis. This colitis was observed to be

21

communicable to genetically intact mice, suggesting loss of T-bet influences bacterial populations to become colitogenic (Garrett et al., 2007). Symbiosis of commensal microorganisms contributes to intestinal immunological homeostasis and protection from pathogens. In the other hand, dysbiosis of commensal bacteria induces abnormal immune responses and causes intestinal inflammation. Now a days metagenomic techniques, makes it possible to retrieve components of microbiota that have co-existed in single donors who have physiologic or disease phenotypes of interest (Goodman et al., 2011). Human micro biome data analysis might be useful for diagnosis and prediction or prognosis of IBD. IBD may be caused by environmental factors, in genetically susceptible individuals, leading to the abnormal host immune responses. Papa et al. have used 16S rRNA sequencing analysis of fecal sample to diagnose pediatric IBD (Papa et al., 2012). Anderson et al. have reported that the patients receiving fecal micro biota transplantation for management of their IBD, has the potential to be an effective and safe treatment for IBD (Anderson et al., 2012).

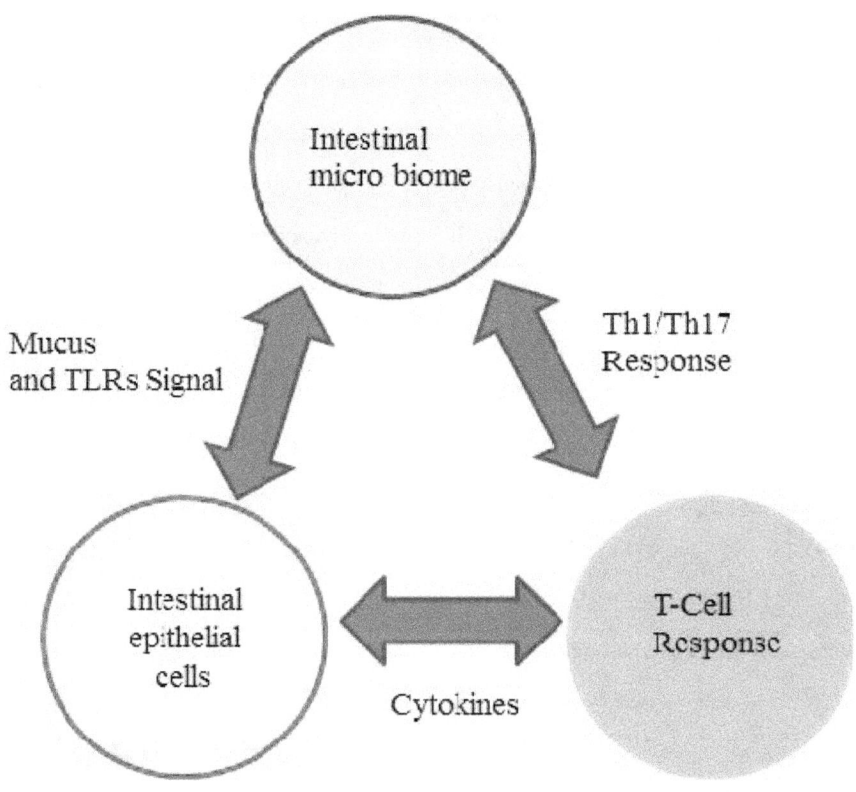

Figure. Gut Immune Homeostasis.

T cell response and epithelial permeability:

Intestinal epithelial cells (IECs) inhibit invasion by pathogens. IECs provide protection through mucus layer covering the surface of the intestinal lumen. Toll-like receptors (TLRs) present on the IECs act like as sensors to recruit immune cells through the production of pro-inflammatory cytokines and also affect epithelial integrity. It has been reported that IEC integrity by claudin 2 up-regulation through PI3 kinase andMyD88 pathways through the activation of TLR2 signaling (Cario et al., 2007). Tight junction proteins like claudin exhibited altered expression level of IECs in Crohn's disease, it may cause increased permeability and bacterial translocation (Zeissig et al., 2007). Cytokine IL-22 has been reported to up regulate the expression of STAT3-dependent molecules (Sugimoto et al., 2008). Recent studies have shown that ILCs (Innate Lymphoid Cells) is produced by IL-22, which modulate the barrier function of IECs (Spits & Di Santo, 2011). Nuding et al. have reported that down regulation of mucosal antimicrobial activity (Nuding et al., 2007). Wehkamp et al. reported that antimicrobial activity was decreased in Crohn's disease with a specific decrease of α-defensin production by Paneth cells being observed (Wehkamp et al., 2005). Shi et al. found that MMP-7-deficient mice, which do not produce the mature form of α-defensin, are susceptible to colitis (Shi et al., 2007). Thus, dysregulation of the production of α-defensins produced by Paneth cells, may alters intestinal microbial ecology through the progression of IBD (Salzman et al., 2010). NF-κB signaling in IECs plays an important role in gut immune homeostasis (Nenci et al.). Nenchiet al. reported that mice lacking NEMO (also named IKKγ) in their IECs conditionally developed spontaneous colitis (Nenci et al., 2007). Günther et al. demonstrated that caspase-8 in IECs plays a key role in protecting these cells from TNF-α-induced necroptotic cell death (Gunther et al., 2011). Rimoldi et al. reported that thymic stromal lymphopoietin (TSLP) produced by IECs leads DCs toward a suppressive phenotype (IL-10 production, but no IL-12 production) and suppresses excessive Th-1 immune responses and, importantly, that the production of TSLP by IECs may be decreased in patients with Crohn's disease (Rimoldi et al., 2005).

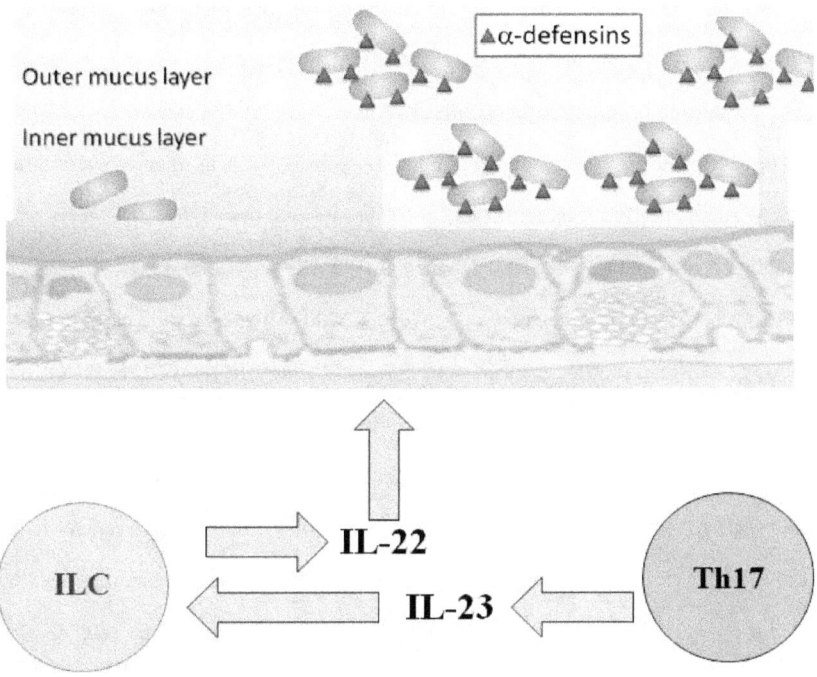

Figure. Th17 Cell response in Intestinal mucosal immunity.

Inflammatory T cells: Th1/ Th17 cells:

Th1 cells develop via a molecular program involving activation of signal transducer and activator of transcription 1 (STAT1) and STAT4, which leads to the induction of T-bet, an essential transcription factor for the development of Th1 cells. T-bet drives the upregulation of IL-12 and acts synergistically with STAT4 to drive optimum expression of IFN-γ (Zhu J, et al.2012). The type I interferons, IL-12 family cytokine and IL-27 contribute to Th1 differentiation through effects on T-bet induction (Takeda A, et al.2003). In Murine models, it has been shown that Th1 cells develop via STAT1 and STAT4 by IFN-γ and IL-12, respectively. IL-17A stimulates several cells including $CD4^+$ memory T lymphocytes to secrete cytokines, resulting in the induction of inflammation (Kolls JK, Linden A.2004). This may play a role in a number of diseases mediated by abnormal immune responses, such as rheumatoid arthritis (Ziolkowska M.2000) and IBD (Fujino S.2003). It has been demonstrated that $CD8^+$ memory T cells, neutrophils and monocytes can also produce IL-17A (Kolls JK.2004). Th17 lineage of $CD4^+$ T cells is a new topic of immunology (Weaver CT., 2006). Th17 cells are categorized by the production of a distinct profile of effector cytokines, including IL-17A, IL-17F, IL-6, IL-22 and IL-26, to enhance host defense responses targeted by Th1 and Th2 cells (Bettelli E., 2007). Th17 cells develop from naive CD4 T cell precursors in the presence of IL-6 and TGF-β, and full differentiation to Th17 cells is dependent on IL-23. Recent studies demonstrated a role for IL-21 in Th17 development (Wilson NJ et al, 2007). IL-21 serves as an autocrine factor secreted by Th17 cells that promotes the Th17 lineage commitment. On the other hand, Th1 cells develop from naive CD4 T cell precursors in the presence of IFN-γ, whereas Th2 cells develop under the control of IL-4. Both IFN-γ and IL-4 inhibit Th17 cell proliferation (Iwakura Y., 2006).

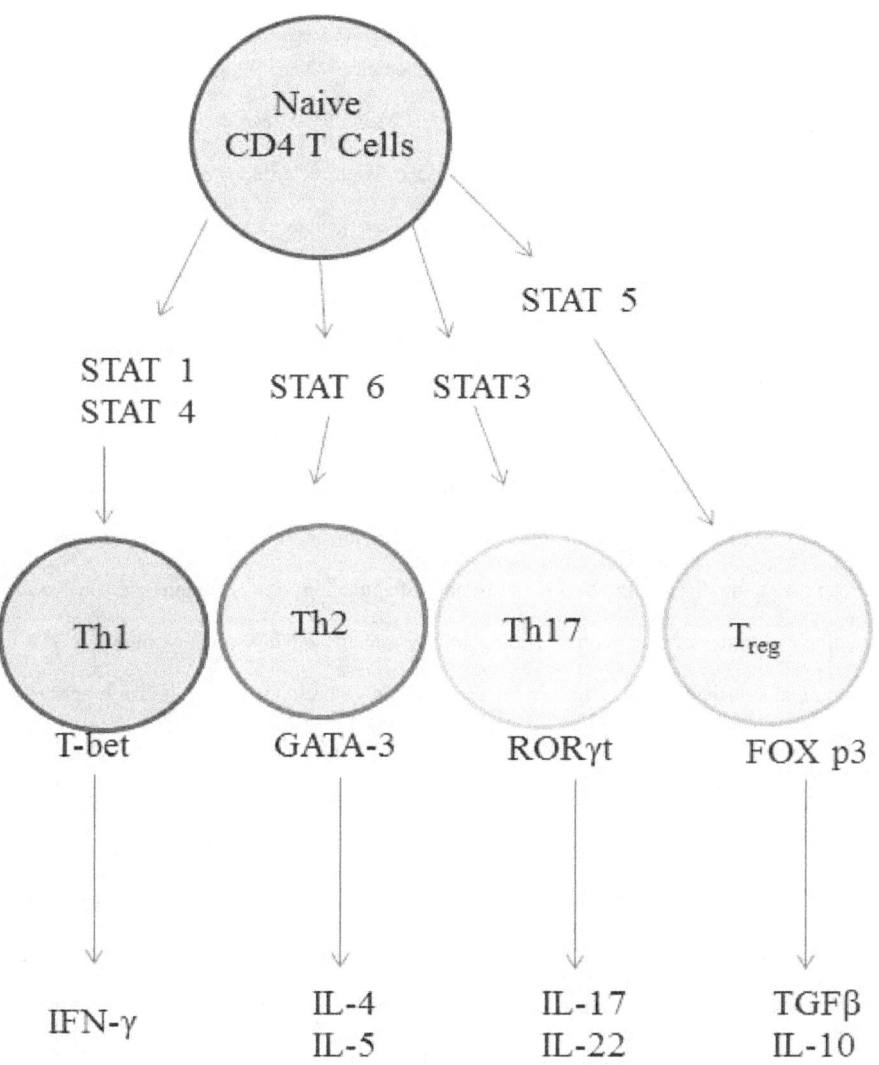

Figure. Differentiation of Th1 and Th17 Cells.

Cytokine and their effector function:

IL-23 modulates Th17 effector function and pathogenicity (Ahern PP, et al., 2010). Th17 cells are involved in homeostasis and inflammation. Th17 cells have been defined by production of IL-17A and the functional characteristics of these cells are determined by the combination of many cytokines. In vitro differentiated cells, and those generated in mice in the absence of specific cytokines involved in Th17 development, suggested significant differences may exist in the pathogenic prospective of the resulting T cells (McGeachy MJ, et al., 2009). A recent study by Vijay Kuchroo et al. (Lee Y, et al., 2012) recognized TGF-β3 as a novel target of IL-23 in CD4$^+$ T cells. TGF-β3, mainly produced by Th17 cells in response to IL-23, drives a distinctive transcriptional signature in Th17 cells. Although, the role of TGF-β3 in intestinal inflammation is currently unclear, the important question of the relationship of intestinal steady-state Th17 cells to those implicated in driving intestinal inflammation clearly requires further study, including definition of their corresponding transcriptional and functional attributes. STAT1 mutations is associated with a disease seen in patients with circulating neutralizing antibodies against key effector cytokines of the Th17 including IL-17A, IL-17F, and IL-22 (Puel A, et al.,2010). Together, these data indicate that Th17 cells are an important component of host defense at mucosal surfaces including the intestine. In human CD, Th17-associated molecules such as IL-17A, IL-17F, IL-21, IL-22, and IL- 23R are increased compared with controls (Brand S., 2009). In mice receiving Wild Type T cells, significant elevation in multiple Th17 cytokines was observed in the intestinal mucosa. By allowing the transfer of T cells deficient in individual cytokines, this model is a particularly elegant system in which the specific role of CD4$^+$ T-cell-derived cytokines in intestinal inflammation can be examined. Using this approach, multiple groups have now demonstrated that T cells deficient in IL-17A are unimpaired in their ability to drive both the intestinal and systemic features of this model (Leppkes M, et al., 2009). In

28

contrast, disease induced by Treg-specific STAT3 deficiency was significantly attenuated by anti-IL- 17A treatment indicating a pathogenic role in some settings (Chaudhry A, et al.,2009).IL-22 is produced by Th17 cells as well as other T cells and appears to have an IL-23 dependency (Sonnenberg GF., 2011).

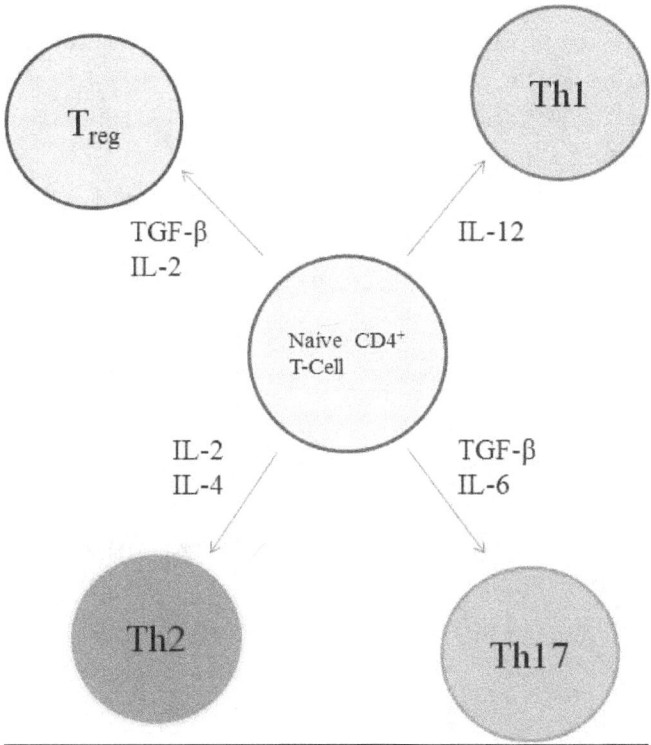

Figure. Role of Cytokines in the T-Cell Differentiation.

References:

Backhed F, Ley RE, Sonnenburg JL, Peterson DA, Gordon JI. Host-bacterial mutualism in the human intestine. Science 2005;307:1915-20.

Kaser A, Zeissig S, Blumberg RS. Inflammatory bowel disease. Annu Rev Immunol 2010;28:573–621.

Elson CO, Cong Y, McCracken VJ, Dimmitt RA, Lorenz RG, Weaver CT. Experimental models of inflammatory bowel disease reveal innate, adaptive, and regulatory mechanisms of host dialogue with the microbiota. Immunol Rev 2005;206: 260-76.

Fujino S, Andoh A, Bamba S, et al. Increased expression of interleukin 17 in inflammatory bowel disease. Gut 2003;52: 65-70.

Fuss IJ, Heller F, Boirivant M, et al. Nonclassical CD1d-restricted NK T cells that produce IL-13 characterize an atypical Th2 response in ulcerative colitis. J Clin Invest 2004;113:1490-7.

Barrett JC, Hansoul S, Nicolae DL, et al. Genome-wide association defines more than 30 distinct susceptibility loci for Crohn's disease. Nat Genet 2008;40:955- 62.

Kullberg MC, et al. Helicobacter hepaticusinduced colitis in interleukin-10-deficient mice: cytokine requirements for the induction and maintenance of intestinal inflammation. Infect Immun 2001;69:4232–4241.

Ahern PP, et al. Interleukin-23 drives intestinal inflammation through direct activity on T cells.Immunity 2010;33:279–288.

Huh JR, et al. Digoxin and its derivatives suppress TH17 cell differentiation by antagonizing RORgammat activity. Nature 2011;472:486–490.

Esplugues E, et al. Control of TH17 cells occurs in the small intestine. Nature 2011;475:514–518.

Ghoreschi K, et al. Generation of pathogenic T (H)17 cells in the absence of TGF-beta signalling. Nature 2010;467:967–971.

McGeachy MJ, et al. The interleukin 23 receptor is essential for the terminal differentiation of interleukin 17-producing effector T helper cells in vivo. Nat Immunol 2009;10:314–324.

Lee Y, et al. Induction and molecular signature of pathogenic TH17 cells. Nat Immunol 2012;13:991–999.

Puel A, et al. Autoantibodies against IL-17A, IL- 17F, and IL-22 in patients with chronic mucocutaneous candidiasis and autoimmune polyendocrine syndrome type I. J Exp Med 2010;207:291–297.

Leppkes M, et al. RORgamma-expressing Th17 cells induce murine chronic intestinal inflammation via redundant effects of IL-17A and IL-17F. Gastroenterology 2009;136:257–267.

Chaudhry A, et al. CD4 + regulatory T cells control TH17 responses in a Stat3-dependent manner. Science 2009;326:986–991.

Sonnenberg GF, Fouser LA, Artis D. Border patrol: regulation of immunity, inflammation and tissue homeostasis at barrier surfaces by IL- 22. Nat Immunol 2011;12:383–390.

Brand S, et al. IL-22 is increased in active Crohn's disease and promotes proinflammatory gene expression and intestinal epithelial cell migration. Am J Physiol Gastrointest Liver Physiol 2006;290:G827–G838.

Broadhurst MJ, et al. IL-22 + CD4 + T cells are associated with therapeutic trichuris trichiura infection in an ulcerative colitis patient. Sci Transl Med 2010;2:60–88.

Korn T, et al. IL-17 and Th17 Cells. Annu Rev Immunol 2009;27:485–517.

R. H. Duerr, K. D. Taylor, S. R. Brant, et al., "A genome-wide association study identifies IL23R as an inflammatory bowel disease gene," *Science*, vol. 314, no. 5804, pp. 1461–1463, 2006.

H. Ito, M. Takazoe, Y. Fukuda, et al., "A pilot randomized trial of a human Anti- interleukin-6 receptor monoclonal antibody in active Crohn's disease," *Gastroenterology*, vol. 126, no. 4, pp. 989–996, 2004.

E. Bettelli, Y. Carrier,W. Gao, et al., "Reciprocal developmental pathways for the generation of pathogenic effector TH17 and regulatory T cells," *Nature*, vol. 441, no. 7090, pp. 235–238, 2006.

Zhu J, et al. The transcription factor T-bet is induced by multiple pathways and prevents an endogenous Th2 cell program during Th1 cell responses. Immunity 2012;37:660–673.

Takeda A, et al. Cutting edge: role of IL-27/ WSX-1 signaling for induction of T-bet through activation of STAT1 during initial Th1 commitment. J Immunol 2003;170:4886–4890.

Kullberg MC, et al. Helicobacter hepaticus triggers colitis in specific-pathogen-free interleukin-10 (IL-10)-deficient mice through an IL-12- and gamma interferon-dependent mechanism. Infect Immun 1998;66:5157–5166.

Simpson SJ, et al. T cell-mediated pathology in two models of experimental colitis depends predominantly on the interleukin 12/Signal transducer and activator of transcription (Stat)-4 pathway, but is not conditional on interferon gamma expression by T cells. J Exp Med 1998;187:1225–1234.

Neurath MF, et al. The transcription factor T-bet regulates mucosal T cell activation in experimental colitis and Crohn's disease. J Exp Med 2002;195:1129–1143.

Rouvier E, Luciani MF, Mattei MG, Denizot F, Golstein P. CTLA-8, cloned from an activated T cell, bearing AU-rich messenger RNA instability sequences, and homologous to a herpesvirus saimiri gene. *J Immunol* 1993; 150: 5445-5456

Kolls JK, Linden A. Interleukin-17 family members and inflammation. *Immunity* 2004; 21: 467-476

Ziolkowska M, Koc A, Luszczykiewicz G, Ksiezopolska- Pietrzak K, Klimczak E, Chwalinska-Sadowska H, Maslinski W. High levels of IL-17 in rheumatoid arthritis patients: IL-15 triggers in vitro IL-17 production via cyclosporine A-sensitive mechanism. *J Immunol* 2000; 164: 2832-2838

Fujino S, Andoh A, Bamba S, Ogawa A, Hata K, Araki Y, Bamba T, Fujiyama Y. Increased expression of interleukin 17 in inflammatory bowel disease. *Gut* 2003; 52: 65-70

Weaver CT, Harrington LE, Mangan PR, Gavrieli M, Murphy KM. Th17: an effector CD4 T cell lineage with regulatory T cell ties. *Immunity* 2006; 24: 677-688

Bettelli E, Korn T, Kuchroo VK. Th17: the third member of the effector T cell trilogy. *Curr Opin Immunol* 2007; 19: 652-657

Wi l son NJ , Boni fac e K, Chan JR, McKenzi e BS, Blumenschein WM, Mattson JD, Basham B, Smith K, Chen T, Morel F, Lecron JC, Kastelein RA, Cua DJ, McClanahanTK, Bowman EP, de Waal Malefyt R. Development, cytokine profile and function of human interleukin 17-producing helper T cells. *Nat Immunol* 2007; 8: 950-957.

Iwakura Y, Ishigame H. The IL-23/IL-17 axis in inflammation. *J Clin Invest* 2006; 116: 1218-1222

Amadi-Obi A, Yu CR, Liu X, Mahdi RM, Clarke GL, Nussenblatt RB, Gery I, Lee YS, Egwuagu CE. TH17 cells contribute to uveitis and scleritis and are expanded by IL-2 and inhibited by IL-27/STAT1. *Nat Med* 2007; 13: 711-718

Cario, E., Gerken, G., & Podolsky, D. K. (2007). Toll-like receptor 2 controls mucosal inflammation by regulating epithelial barrier function. Gastroenterology 132, 1359–1374.

Zeissig, S., Burgel, N., Gunzel, D., Richter, J., Mankertz, J., Wahnschaffe, U., et al. (2007). Changes in expression and distribution of claudin 2, 5 and 8 lead to discontinuous tight junctions and barrier dysfunction in active Crohn's disease. Gut 56, 61–72.

Sugimoto, K., Ogawa, A., Mizoguchi, E., Shimomura, Y., Andoh, A., Bhan, A. K., et al. (2008). IL-22 ameliorates intestinal inflammation in a mouse model of ulcerative colitis. J Clin Invest 118, 534–544.

Spits, H., & Di Santo, J. P. (2011). The expanding family of innate lymphoid cells: Regulators and effectors of immunity and tissue remodeling. Nat Immunol 12, 21–27.

Nuding, S., Fellermann, K., Wehkamp, J., & Stange, E. F. (2007). Reduced mucosal antimicrobial activity in Crohn's disease of the colon. Gut 56, 1240–1247.

Wehkamp, J., Salzman, N. H., Porter, E., Nuding, S., Weichenthal, M., Petras, R. E., et al. (2005). Reduced Paneth cell alpha-defensins in ileal Crohn's disease. Proc Natl Acad Sci U S A 102, 18129–18134.

Tanabe, H., Ayabe, T., Maemoto, A., Ishikawa, C., Inaba, Y., Sato, R., et al. (2007). Denatured human alpha-defensin attenuates the bactericidal activity and the stability against enzymatic digestion. Biochem Biophys Res Commun 358, 349–355.

Shi, J., Aono, S., Lu, W., Ouellette, A. J., Hu, X., Ji, Y., et al. (2007). A novel role for defensins in intestinal homeostasis: Regulation of IL-1beta secretion. J Immunol 179, 1245–1253.

Salzman, N. H., Hung, K., Haribhai, D., Chu, H., Karlsson-Sjoberg, J., Amir, E., et al. (2010). Enteric defensins are essential regulators of intestinal microbial ecology. Nat Immunol 11, 76–83.

Nenci, A., Becker, C., Wullaert, A., Gareus, R., van Loo, G., Danese, S., et al. (2007). Epithelial NEMO links innate immunity to chronic intestinal inflammation. Nature ,446, 557–561.

Gunther, C., Martini, E., Wittkopf, N., Amann, K., Weigmann, B., Neumann, H., et al. (2011). Caspase-8 regulates TNF-alpha-induced epithelial necroptosis and terminal ileitis. Nature 477, 335–339.

Rimoldi, M., Chieppa, M., Salucci, V., Avogadri, F., Sonzogni, A., Sampietro, G. M., et al. (2005). Intestinal immune homeostasis is regulated by the crosstalk between epithelial cells and dendritic cells. Nat Immunol 6, 507–514.

Stockinger, B., & Veldhoen, M. (2007). Differentiation and function of Th17 T cells. Curr Opin Immunol 19, 281–286.

Atarashi, K., Tanoue, T., Shima, T., Imaoka, A., Kuwahara, T., Momose, Y., et al. (2011). Induction of colonic regulatory T cells by indigenous Clostridium species. Science 331, 337–341.

Mazmanian, S. K., Round, J. L., & Kasper, D. L. (2008). A microbial symbiosis factor prevents intestinal inflammatory disease. Nature 453, 620–625.

Round, J. L., & Mazmanian, S. K. (2010). Inducible Foxp3+regulatory T-cell development by a commensal bacterium of the intestinal microbiota. Proc Natl Acad Sci U S A 107, 12204–12209.

Barrett, J. C., Hansoul, S., Nicolae, D. L., Cho, J. H., Duerr, R. H., Rioux, J. D., et al. (2008). Genome-wide association defines more than 30 distinct susceptibility loci for Crohn's disease. Nat Genet 40, 955–962.

Garrett, W. S., Lord, G. M., Punit, S., Lugo-Villarino, G., Mazmanian, S. K., Ito, S., et al. (2007). Communicable ulcerative colitis induced by T-bet deficiency in the innate immune system. Cell 131, 33–45.

Goodman, A. L., Kallstrom, G., Faith, J. J., Reyes, A., Moore, A., Dantas, G., et al. (2011). Extensive personal human gut microbiota culture collections characterized and manipulated in gnotobiotic mice. Proc Natl Acad Sci U S A 108, 6252–6257.

Papa, E., Docktor, M., Smillie, C., Weber, S., Preheim, S. P., Gevers, D., et al. (2012). Noninvasive mapping of the gastrointestinal microbiota identifies children with inflammatory bowel disease. PLoS One 7, e39242.

Anderson, J. L., Edney, R. J., & Whelan, K. (2012). Systematic review: Faecal microbiota transplantation in the management of inflammatory bowel disease. Aliment Pharmacol Ther 36, 503–516.

Barnes MJ, Powrie F. Regulatory T cells reinforce intestinal homeostasis. Immunity 2009;31: 401–411.

Saraiva M, O'Garra A. The regulation of IL-10 production by immune cells. Nat Rev Immunol 2010;10:170–181.

Barnes MJ, Powrie F. Regulatory T cells reinforce intestinal homeostasis. Immunity 2009;31: 401–411.

Davidson NJ, et al. T helper cell 1-type CD4 + T cells, but not B cells, mediate colitis in interleukin 10-deficient mice. J Exp Med 1996;184:241–251.

Moore KW, et al. Interleukin-10 and the interleukin-10 receptor. Annu Rev Immunol 2001;19:683–765.

Chaudhry A, et al. Interleukin-10 signaling in regulatory T cells is required for suppression of Th17 cell-mediated inflammation. Immunity 2011;34:566–578.

Chaudhry A, et al. CD4 + regulatory T cells control TH17 responses in a Stat3-dependent manner. Science 2009;326:986–991.

Glocker EO, et al. IL-10 and IL-10 receptor defects in humans. Ann NY Acad Sci 2011;1246:102–107.

Maloy KJ, Powrie F. Intestinal homeostasis and its breakdown in inflammatory bowel disease. Nature 2011;474:298–306.

Wildin RS, et al. X-linked neonatal diabetes mellitus, enteropathy and endocrinopathy syndrome is the human equivalent of mouse scurfy. Nat Genet 2001;27:18–20.

Josefowicz SZ, Lu LZ, Rudensky AY. Regulatory T cells: mechanisms of differentiation and function. Annu Rev Immunol 2012;30:531–564.

Haribhai D, et al. A central role for induced regulatory T cells in tolerance induction in experimental colitis. J Immunol 2009;182: 3461–3468.

Weiss JM, et al. Neuropilin 1 is expressed on thymus-derived natural regulatory T cells, but not mucosa-generated induced Foxp3 + T reg cells. J Exp Med 2012;209:1723–1742.

Zheng Y, et al. Role of conserved non-coding DNA elements in the Foxp3 gene in regulatory T-cell fate. Nature 2010;463:808–812.

Josefowicz SZ, et al. Extrathymically generated regulatory T cells control mucosal TH2 inflammation. Nature 2012;482:395–399.

Haribhai D, et al. A requisite role for induced regulatory T cells in tolerance based on expanding antigen receptor diversity. Immunity 2011;35:109–122.

Haribhai D, et al. A central role for induced regulatory T cells in tolerance induction in experimental colitis. J Immunol 2009;182: 3461–3468.

Lathrop SK, et al. Antigen-specific peripheral shaping of the natural regulatory T cell population. J Exp Med 2008;205:3105–3117.

Lathrop SK, et al. Peripheral education of the immune system by colonic commensal microbiota. Nature 2011;478:250–254.

Publisher: Eliva Press SRL

Email: info@elivapress.com

Eliva Press is an independent publishing house established for the publication and dissemination of academic works all over the world. Company provides high quality and professional service for all of our authors.

Our Services:
Free of charge, open-minded, eco-friendly, innovational.

-Free standard publishing services (manuscript review, step-by-step book preparation, publication, distribution, and marketing).
-No financial risk. The author is not obliged to pay any hidden fees for publication.
-Editors. Dedicated editors will assist step by step through the projects.
-Money paid to the author for every book sold. Up to 50% royalties guaranteed.
-ISBN (International Standard Book Number). We assign a unique ISBN to every Eliva Press book.
-Digital archive storage. Books will be available online for a long time. We don't need to have a stock of our titles. No unsold copies. Eliva Press uses environment friendly print on demand technology that limits the needs of publishing business. We care about environment and share these principles with our customers.
-Cover design. Cover art is designed by a professional designer.
-Worldwide distribution. We continue expanding our distribution channels to make sure that all readers have access to our books.

www.ingramcontent.com/pod-product-compliance
Lightning Source LLC
Chambersburg PA
CBHW051300170526
45165CB00004B/1784